NCCN Guidelines for Patients®

The essential guide for people facing cancer.

Based on care recommendations from leading cancer experts.

Explains high-quality cancer care provided at state-of-the-art cancer centers.

Reviewed and revised every year.

Did you know that top cancer centers across the United States work together to improve cancer care? This alliance of leading cancer centers is called the National Comprehensive Cancer Network® (NCCN®).

Because cancer care is always evolving, NCCN develops and frequently updates evidence-based cancer care recommendations used by health care providers worldwide. These recommendations are known as the NCCN Clinical Practice Guidelines in Oncology (NCCN Guidelines®).

The NCCN Guidelines for Patients plainly explain these expert recommendations, so you can talk with your care team about the best care for you.

These NCCN Guidelines for Patients are based on the NCCN Guidelines® for Hematopoietic Growth Factors, Version 3.2026 – December 5, 2025.

View the NCCN Guidelines for Patients free online: NCCN.org/patientguidelines

Find an NCCN Cancer Center near you: NCCN.org/cancercenters

Learn how the NCCN Guidelines for Patients are developed: NCCN.org/patient-guidelines-process

Connect with us

@NCCNorg @NCCNVideo NCCN @NCCNorg

Supporters

NCCN Guidelines for Patients are supported by funding from the NCCN Foundation®

To make a gift, visit NCCNFoundation.org/Donate

To learn more, visit online NCCN.org/patientguidelines or email PatientGuidelines@NCCN.org

Contents

NCCN Foundation seeks to support the millions of patients and their families affected by a cancer diagnosis by funding and distributing NCCN Guidelines for Patients. NCCN Foundation is also committed to advancing cancer treatment by funding the nation's promising doctors at the center of innovation in cancer research. For more details and the full library of patient and caregiver resources, visit NCCN.org/patients.

National Comprehensive Cancer Network (NCCN) and NCCN Foundation
3025 Chemical Road, Suite 100, Plymouth Meeting, PA 19462 USA

1
About low blood cell counts

If you're undergoing cancer treatment, you may develop low blood cell counts. This can be upsetting and can cause health problems. This chapter explains low blood cell counts.

What are low blood cell counts?

Low blood cell counts can happen when you have specific cancers, conditions, or treatments.

This can restrict the amount of healthy red blood cells, white blood cells, and platelets in your bloodstream. Low blood counts can result in health problems.

Low blood cell counts are also called:

- **Anemia** (uh-NEE-me-YUH) is a low red blood cell count
- **Neutropenia** (new-tro-PEEN-ee-ya) is a low white blood cell count
- **Thrombocytopenia** (throm-BO-site-TOH-PEEN-ee-ya) is a low platelet count

This guide describes each of these types of low blood counts and provides NCCN expert guidelines and recommendations for treatment.

How this guide can help you

Making decisions about cancer care is stressful. There's a lot to learn, and you don't know what the future holds.

Use this guide to get the information and support you need.

Patients, doctors, and other health care professionals trust the NCCN Guidelines for Patients. This guide uses clear, everyday language to explain current cancer care recommendations made by respected experts in the field. Their recommendations are based on the latest research and practices at leading cancer centers.

Your health is unique to you, so your cancer care should be, too. As you read this guide, you'll learn which treatments are likely to provide the best results for you. And you'll be better prepared to talk with your care team.

Anemia

Anemia is when the body has a lack of red blood cells. Red blood cells carry oxygen from the lungs to the rest of the body.

Red blood cells look like tiny, flat doughnuts without holes. They get their red color from hemoglobin, a protein that picks up oxygen in the lungs.

As the blood travels throughout the body, hemoglobin delivers oxygen to different body parts. In exchange, red blood cells receive carbon dioxide from tissues and organs and carry it back into the lungs, where you breathe it out.

The signs and symptoms of anemia include:

- Pale skin
- Shortness of breath
- Heart palpitations, or a fluttering sensation in your chest
- Heart murmurs
- Feeling sluggish or slow to move
- Fatigue

Healthy red blood cells live for 3 months until they're replaced.

Neutropenia

Neutropenia means there's a low level of white blood cells in the body. White blood cells are important to the immune system because they fight infections.

For example, bacteria or a virus can enter your blood through a cut in your skin. Once the body detects the invading germ, white blood cells surround and destroy it.

But neutropenia lowers your immune system's defenses and raises your risk for infection.

Neutropenia itself doesn't cause symptoms. Symptoms come from infections that occur as a result of neutropenia.

Signs and symptoms include:

- Frequent infections
- Fever
- Swollen glands in the throat or armpit
- Mouth sores
- Rash
- Fatigue
- Diarrhea

You can also have neutropenia without any symptoms.

Healthy white blood cells live for 8 to 14 days, until they're replaced.

Thrombocytopenia

Thrombocytopenia happens when the body's platelet count is low. Platelets clump together to stop bleeding. If your platelet count is too low, you may have unnecessary or unusual bleeding.

Platelets are tiny, plate-shaped cells. Platelets work to control bleeding inside your body and on your skin. For example, when a blood vessel is damaged, platelets bind together to create a clot.

The signs and symptoms of thrombocytopenia include:

- Bleeding gums; nosebleeds; or bleeding from the mouth, butt, or injection sites
- Bruising more easily or more severely than usual

- A rash of small, flat, red, purple, or brown spots under the skin, called petechiae, caused by leaking blood vessels
- Bleeding in the skin that can cause red, purple, or brownish-yellow spots called purpura
- Heavy menstrual bleeding or bleeding that lasts longer than normal
- Blood in pee, poop, vomit, or mucus
- Severe headaches or blurred vision

Platelets survive only about 9 days in the bloodstream. New platelets are constantly replacing older ones.

What is ICAHT?

ICAHT (also known as immune effector cell-associated hematotoxicity) is a life-threatening side effect of some cancer treatments, including chimeric antigen receptor (CAR) T-cell therapies. With ICAHT, a person can have neutropenia, anemia, and thrombocytopenia all at once.

This guide has the latest NCCN guidelines for treating and preventing ICAHT, and you'll learn more in *Chapter 6: ICAHT and supportive care*.

How are low blood cell counts managed?

Treatment for any low blood cell count involves replacing the cells that are missing, either with donor blood or through stimulating the body to create more.

Treatment for each type of low blood cell count is described in detail in *Chapter 3: Treating anemia, Chapter 4: Treating neutropenia, and Chapter 5: Treating thrombocytopenia*.

How can I get the best care?

Advocate for yourself. You have an important role to play in your care. Many people feel more satisfied when they actively take part in planning their cancer care.

The NCCN Guidelines for Patients will help you play a larger role in your care. Discuss the recommendations in this guide with your care team. Ask questions about your options and share your goals and concerns.

Don't know what to ask? You're not alone. That's why we include suggested questions to ask at the end of chapters.

Keep reading to find the best care for you.

2

Testing for low blood cell counts

You may have frequent blood tests to figure out the cause of low blood cell counts. Low blood cell counts don't always cause obvious symptoms.

If you're undergoing cancer treatment, you'll need to have blood tests regularly in addition to the standard health tests that everyone gets. Blood tests are done by placing a needle into your arm and taking a sample of blood. Your blood is then tested in a lab.

If you know your veins are difficult to find, let the lab tech know and they can get a machine that will help find your veins. This way, you'll get fewer pokes from the needle, and it's less stressful.

Blood tests

Complete blood count with indices

A complete blood count with indices measures the number and physical makeup of cells in the blood.

Guide 1
Tests for low blood counts

Needed tests	Complete blood count (CBC) with indices
	Blood smear morphology
	Reticulocyte count
	Imaging test(s) of the chest, abdomen, and pelvis
Tests used in some cases	Hemolysis testing
	Nutritional testing
	Family history
	Renal dysfunction testing
	Treatment-induced myelosuppression
	Hormone dysfunction testing
	Anemia of chronic inflammation
	Medical history

Your doctor will be specifically interested in your blood's hematocrit and hemoglobin levels.

A hematocrit test checks the percentage of red blood cells in the blood. Hemoglobin helps move oxygen around the body, so when there's a low amount, it could indicate low blood counts.

A low hematocrit or hemoglobin count is a sign of anemia.

If your results indicate low blood cell counts, such as anemia, neutropenia, or thrombocytopenia, your doctor may ask for further blood testing, including a blood smear test.

Blood smear

A blood smear is a test for abnormal blood cells. It examines both red and white blood cells. The blood smear helps define the shape of red blood cells and the presence of abnormal cells. These abnormal blood cells can prevent healthy blood cells from doing their jobs.

If the blood smear finds abnormal cells, further testing may be necessary to determine if they're caused by cancer or organ damage.

Reticulocyte count

A reticulocyte is a young red blood cell. This test helps to determine the cause and type of anemia by counting the number of young red blood cells in the blood. The test shows whether your bone marrow is making red blood cells at a normal rate. If it's higher or lower than normal, you may have bone marrow dysfunction, certain types of cancer, or vitamin deficiencies.

Mean corpuscular volume

Mean corpuscular volume measures the average size of red blood cells. This test is especially helpful in identifying iron-deficiency anemia.

In iron-deficiency anemia, red blood cells tend to be smaller than normal (microcytic). Other types of anemia, such as macrocytic anemia, are caused by larger-than-normal blood cells.

Nutritional tests

Nutritional tests check for chemicals in your blood that can also be found in things you eat. These are still blood tests, but they check for the levels of these chemicals.

The test is performed by drawing a blood sample and sending it to a lab to be tested.

Iron

Aside from being a nutritional necessity found in leafy greens and meat, iron is an important component of hemoglobin in the blood. As mentioned before, hemoglobin is essential in the breathing cycle because it moves oxygen around in the bloodstream.

An iron test may be performed if your doctor suspects too little iron (deficiency) or too much iron (overload). Either can be an indication of anemia.

Total iron-binding capacity

A total iron-binding capacity test is used to see how well transferrin, which transports iron through your blood, is doing its job. Transferrin is created in the liver.

A lower-than-normal total iron-binding capacity could indicate liver damage or nutrition problems. A higher-than-normal result usually means you have iron-deficiency anemia.

Ferritin

Ferritin is a protein in the blood that contains iron. A ferritin test is used to find out how much iron is stored in your body.

If a ferritin test result shows lower-than-normal results, you may have iron-deficiency anemia. If the test results show a higher-than-normal rate, this can indicate swelling and inflammation, which can be a sign of liver, spleen, or bone marrow damage.

Vitamin B12 and folate

Vitamin B12 and folate are nutrients only found in the food you eat. Vitamin B12 and folate tests measure vitamin levels in the liquid portion of the blood to detect deficiencies. Deficiencies in vitamin B12 and folate can cause extreme tiredness, or fatigue.

Testing for hemolytic anemia

Healthy hemolysis is when red blood cells are broken down. This can happen in a few different ways, for example, from infections or medications like aspirin.

In hemolytic anemia, your red blood cells are destroyed faster than your bone marrow can make new red blood cells. This results in a shortage of healthy red blood cells.

If you might have hemolytic anemia, your health care provider may request a test of one of these substances:

- Direct antiglobulin
- Haptoglobin
- Bilirubin
- Lactate dehydrogenase

Hemolysis

Hemolysis is a rupture or destruction of red blood cells.

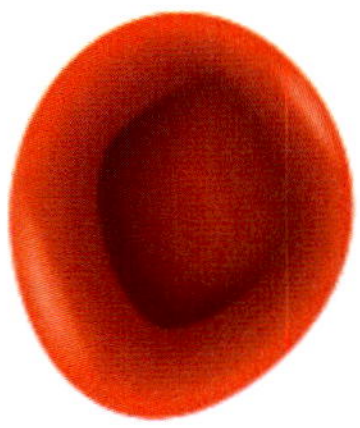

Normal red blood cell (erythrocyte)

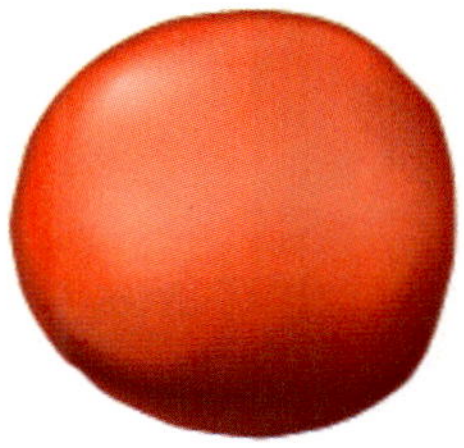

Spherocyte (erythrocytes that are sphere shaped)

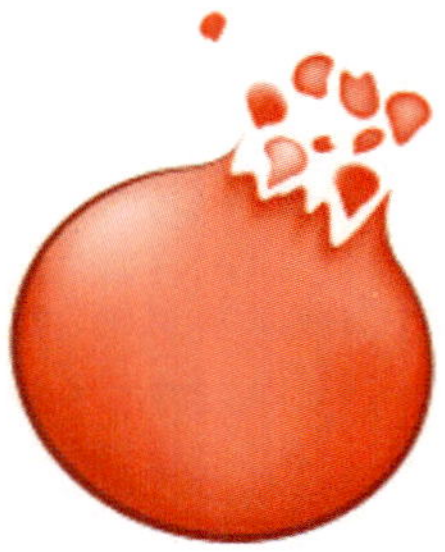

Rupturing of erythrocyte and the release of contents into blood plasma

Direct antiglobulin

Hemolytic anemia stimulates your immune system to make germ-fighting cells (antibodies) that mistakenly attack your red blood cells. If a direct antiglobulin test finds these antibodies in your blood, it confirms you have hemolytic anemia.

Haptoglobin

A haptoglobin test measures the amount of haptoglobin in your blood. It's a protein that binds with hemoglobin to help transport oxygen. Haptoglobin also helps prevent hemolysis.

A lower-than-normal haptoglobin result means that your blood is more prone to hemolysis-causing conditions like hemolytic anemia.

Bilirubin

Bilirubin is a yellowish pigment created during the breakdown of red blood cells. A bilirubin test measures the levels of bilirubin in your blood.

Higher-than-normal bilirubin levels can be caused by an increased rate of destruction of red blood cells, which can be a sign of hemolytic anemia.

Lactate dehydrogenase

Lactate dehydrogenase can be used to measure how well cancer medicine works. It's found in many organs and tissues in the body, including the liver, heart, pancreas, kidneys, skeletal muscles, lymph tissue, and blood cells.

A lactate dehydrogenase test is used to see if you have any tissue damage.

Kidney testing for anemia

These blood tests measure how the kidneys can be involved in low blood counts, particularly anemia.

Glomerular filtration rate

Glomeruli are tiny filters in the kidneys that clean out waste from the blood. Glomerular filtration rate is a blood test used to estimate how much blood passes through the glomeruli each minute.

If the glomerular filtration rate is lower than average, that can mean anemia. When the glomeruli aren't filtering the blood properly, then less of the chemical needed to make blood cells (erythropoietin) will be produced, resulting in lower red blood cell counts.

Creatinine

Creatinine is a waste product created in the muscles. It can also be tested in a blood sample.

Higher-than-average creatinine levels can mean your kidneys are impaired and cannot filter the blood well. If this is the case, then it can cause anemia.

Testing for neutropenia

C-reactive protein

C-reactive protein, or CRP, is found in the liquid portion of the blood. CRP increases when there's inflammation in your body.

A CRP test is used to check for increased inflammation. Inflammation can indicate neutropenia, because a lower white blood cell count can lead to more infections and inflammation.

Erythrocyte sedimentation rate

An erythrocyte sedimentation rate is a blood test that measures inflammation, if any, in the bloodstream. Inflammation can indicate infection, which can be a symptom of neutropenia.

Hormone imbalances related to illness

Hormones are messengers that travel through your body to make certain things happen. For example, humans have a hormone called erythropoietin that tells the body to make red blood cells.

When these messengers are kept from doing their jobs, it can cause low blood cell counts.

Hypogonadism

Hypogonadism is a condition where the body unintentionally does not produce enough sex hormones. These hormones include testosterone for those who were assigned male at birth and estrogen for those assigned female at birth.

People with low testosterone levels may have low red blood cell counts. Because of this, you may be tested for low hormone levels. Treatment for hypogonadism may include

Erythrocyte sedimentation rate

This test measures how quickly red blood cells settle at the bottom of the test tube.

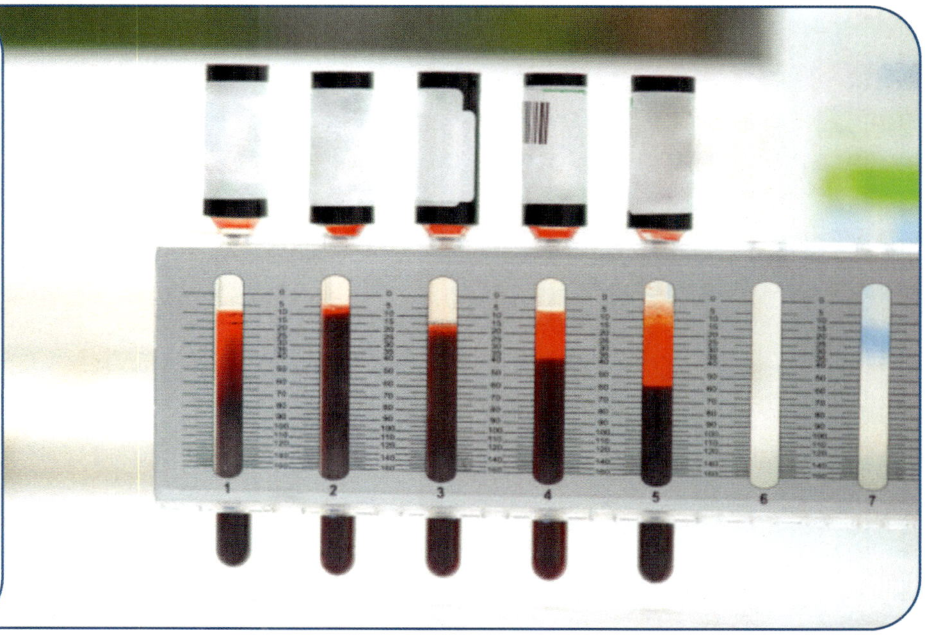

hormone replacement therapy and assisted reproduction.

Adrenal dysfunction

Your adrenal glands are located above the kidneys. Adrenal insufficiency, or Addison's disease, is a disorder where your adrenal glands do not produce enough cortisol and aldosterone. This can cause symptoms of anemia or neutropenia.

Cortisol is released by the adrenal glands to help your body deal with stressful situations. Aldosterone helps to balance sodium and potassium in your blood.

Tests can measure the levels of cortisol and aldosterone in your body. Too much cortisol can lead to higher blood pressure and a heightened feeling of stress. Too much aldosterone can cause you to lose potassium and retain sodium.

General health tests

Family history

Some cancers and other diseases run in families. Your doctor will ask about the health history of family members who are blood relatives. This information is called a family history.

If you can, you should ask family members about their health issues like heart disease, cancer, and diabetes and how old they were when diagnosed.

Health history

A health history is a record of all health issues and treatments you've had in your life.

Be prepared to list any illness or injury and when it happened. Bring a list of old and new medicines and any over-the-counter medicines, herbal remedies, or supplements you take. Your health history will help determine which treatment is best for you.

Physical exam

A member of your care team will perform a thorough physical exam of your body. This exam includes checking vital signs, such as heart rate. Your provider will also look over your body and gently press on certain areas, feeling for anything unusual with your organs or lymph nodes.

Endoscopy

Endoscopy is a non-surgical test that uses a flexible tube with a light and camera to look inside your digestive tract. It allows the care team to ensure you're not bleeding in your stomach. You'll be asleep during this procedure.

Key points

- Doctors use a blood test called a complete blood count to diagnose anemia. A complete blood count measures the number and physical makeup of cells found in your blood.
- Some cancers and other diseases can run in families, so it's important to tell your care team about any family history of disease that you know about.

Questions to ask

- Will any of the tests you're recommending be uncomfortable or painful?
- How can I prepare for testing?
- Will my health insurance pay for these tests?
- My veins are hard to find. Do you have a vein finder?

What's next?

After your tests, you may receive a diagnosis of anemia, neutropenia, or thrombocytopenia. NCCN expert recommendations can guide your treatment plan. To learn more about these recommendations, read on to the next few chapters.

"Adapt your lifestyle (to a better one). Don't be ashamed to be a long sleeper. Take days of rest. Living slower is a luxury. I take it as a gift."

3 Treating anemia

There are many forms of anemia, each with its own cause and symptoms. This chapter focuses on anemia caused by cancer or chemotherapy treatment.

Anemia is a condition where your blood doesn't have enough healthy red blood cells, resulting in less oxygen in your body. If there's less oxygen circulating through your body, you might feel fatigued or lightheaded.

If your anemia is severe, you may be treated with a blood transfusion, iron supplements, or medications to stimulate red blood cell production.

There are many types and causes of anemia. Mild anemia is a common and treatable condition that can occur in anyone.

Anemia may also be a sign of a more serious condition. It may result from chronic bleeding in the stomach, chronic inflammation from an infection, kidney disease, cancer, or an autoimmune disease.

This chapter focuses on anemia caused by cancer and chemotherapy. It also focuses on cancer's relationship with anemia.

Anemia and cancer

Anemia is a very common side effect of chemotherapy. Chemotherapy drugs kill fast-growing cells like cancer and blood cells. Severe anemia caused by chemotherapy may result in a delay in treatments or a need to reduce the chemotherapy dose. Any delay in

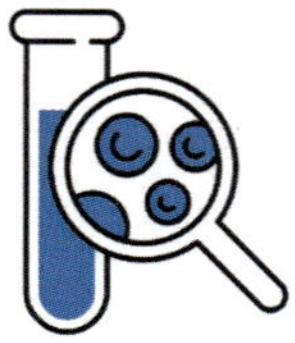

Anemia

Anemia occurs when the body cannot produce enough red blood cells to move oxygen toward tissues and organs.

- Anemia can cause breathing difficulties, cold fingers and toes, pale skin, and frequent headaches.
- Anemia can affect people of all ages, races, and ethnicities. Some types of anemia are very common, and some are very rare.
- Causes of anemia may include blood loss or too few red blood cells. Factors that may cause too few red blood cells include diet, medical conditions, or genetic disorders.
- If the anemia is due to a poor diet, eating more dark, leafy green vegetables; nuts; dried fruit; red meat; grains; citrus fruits; and beans may help.
- Anemia symptoms can also be risk factors for other diseases and disorders. This means the anemia could possibly be overlooked or misdiagnosed.
- Work with your doctor to determine the cause of anemia. You are more likely to stay healthy and avoid other serious health conditions in the long run.

chemotherapy treatments may cause them to be less effective.

Causes of anemia for people with cancer include:

- Chemotherapy drugs
- Bleeding of any kind
- Cancers that destroy the body's ability to make new blood cells

Under healthy conditions, the kidneys produce a hormone to tell the body to make more red blood cells. If the kidneys are damaged from cancer, chemotherapy, or radiation therapy, there won't be enough of the hormone to signal for more red blood cells. This can cause anemia.

How is anemia treated?

Treatment depends on the type of anemia and the cause. Iron supplements may be used to treat iron deficiency. Blood transfusions may be used for blood loss. Certain medications may be used to bump up blood cell production.

Red blood cell transfusion

The fastest way to increase red blood cell counts is with a blood transfusion. This is a routine procedure where donated blood is given to you through a vein in your arm.

A blood transfusion typically takes 1 to 4 hours, depending on how much is needed and what part of the blood you need.

You should expect to receive regular blood tests to test your blood counts before and

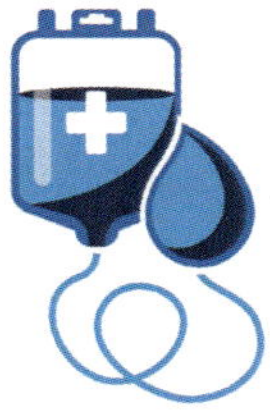

Transfusions

A transfusion is a common procedure to replace blood or blood components (red blood cells or platelets). It is given to you through an intravenous (IV) line, a tiny tube that is inserted into a vein with a small needle.

- The whole process can take about 1 to 4 hours, depending on how much blood is needed.
- Most transfusions use blood from a donor. Some choose a family member or friend to donate blood.
- Blood transfusions are usually very safe. Donated blood is carefully tested, handled, and stored.
- Most people's bodies handle blood transfusions very well. But, like any medical procedure, there are some risks. Speak with your doctor for specific information about your risks.
- Chemotherapy can affect how bone marrow makes new blood cells. Some people getting treatment for cancer might need a transfusion of red blood cells or platelets.

after transfusions. Sometimes, you may need more than one blood transfusion.

Before your first blood transfusion, you'll be evaluated to see how severe the anemia is. If you are not experiencing symptoms and don't have other major health issues, no treatment is necessary.

If your red blood cell numbers continue to decline due to recent chemotherapy or radiation therapy and you have no other major health issues, your doctor will recommend treatment with a red blood cell transfusion.

If you have symptoms of anemia, you'll be tested for the following health concerns before starting treatment:

- Heart disease or chest pain
- Fast or labored breathing
- Lightheadedness or fainting
- Fatigue

Side effects of red blood cell transfusion

There are risks of side effects from red blood cell transfusion, including:

- Allergic reactions
- Fever
- Infection
- Volume overload
- Too much iron

These side effects tend to be rare.

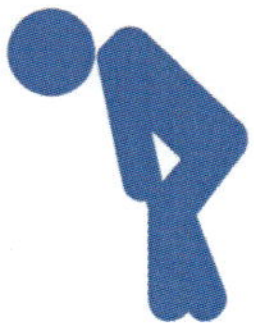

Fatigue

Fatigue is common with cancer. Anemia may make fatigue worse. Anemia can also impact your cancer treatment.

Erythropoietic therapy

Erythropoietin is a hormone made in the kidneys. It boosts the creation of red blood cells.

Erythropoiesis-stimulating agents, or ESAs, are drugs that work like erythropoietin. They are used to treat anemia caused by chemotherapy, chronic kidney disease, or certain treatments for HIV.

ESAs can help reduce the need for blood transfusions during chemotherapy treatment.

Epoetin alfa (Procrit and Epogen) and darbepoetin alfa (Aranesp) are examples of erythropoiesis-stimulating agents. A biosimilar, epoetin alfa-epbx (Retacrit), is also available, which has a similar effect but is made differently.

You may receive ESA treatment if you have anemia and you:

- Are undergoing chemotherapy
- Have chronic kidney disease
- Don't want or cannot have a blood transfusion

ESAs might cause the following conditions:

- An increase in the risk of blood clots in your veins
- Higher risk for heart attack, stroke, heart failure, and death
- Growth of tumor(s) in some people (but typically, the cancer doesn't get worse)

Increasing iron

Iron is an essential mineral that's necessary to maintain healthy cells, skin, hair, and nails. It's also important for producing hemoglobin, the molecule in your blood that carries oxygen through the body.

If your iron levels are low, your health care provider may treat you with an intravenous (IV) iron supplement. Side effects caused by IV iron may include feeling flushed, headaches, and joint or muscle aches days after treatment.

Or, your health care provider may treat you with an oral iron supplement, or a pill. Oral iron is used for less severe iron deficiency but may cause stomach issues.

Key points

- Anemia is a condition where your body does not make enough healthy blood cells, resulting in less oxygen being carried to your cells.
- Severe anemia caused by chemotherapy may delay treatments or reduce your chemotherapy dose.
- The fastest way to treat anemia is with a red blood cell transfusion.
- Erythropoiesis-stimulating agents (ESAs) stimulate the bone marrow to make more red blood cells, which can cause cancer to recur (but not worsen).

Questions to ask

- Are there any treatments that you don't recommend for anemia?
- Do you have access to a compatible blood type for me?

"If it weren't for cancer, I'd say I had a perfect life. If it weren't for cancer, would I even realize this?"

4

Treating neutropenia

Neutropenia refers to a low number of white blood cells. This can lead to an increase in the risk of infections. This chapter presents an overview of neutropenia.

Neutropenia is a low number of white blood cells (neutrophils). White blood cells are important in fighting infection in the body. With fewer germ-fighting white blood cells, your body will be at greater risk for infection.

When neutropenia is severe, even the bacteria normally found in your mouth and intestines can cause a serious illness.

Certain cancers and cancer treatments can cause neutropenia. It's common after receiving chemotherapy. This is because chemotherapy kills cancer cells as well as healthy white blood cells.

Most people aren't aware they have neutropenia because it doesn't cause symptoms on its own. People often find out when they have a blood test performed for other reasons.

How does neutropenia occur?

Neutropenia can occur in a couple of ways. One is that the white blood cells (neutrophils) are used up or destroyed faster than they can be made. The other way is that the bone marrow does not make enough white blood cells.

Neutropenia often occurs between 7 and 12 days after you receive chemotherapy. Timing depends on the type of chemotherapy you receive.

A member of your treatment team will let you know when your white blood cell count is likely to be at its lowest. During this time, you should

Neutropenia

Neutropenia describes a low number of white blood cells called neutrophils. Neutrophils are important in fighting infections.

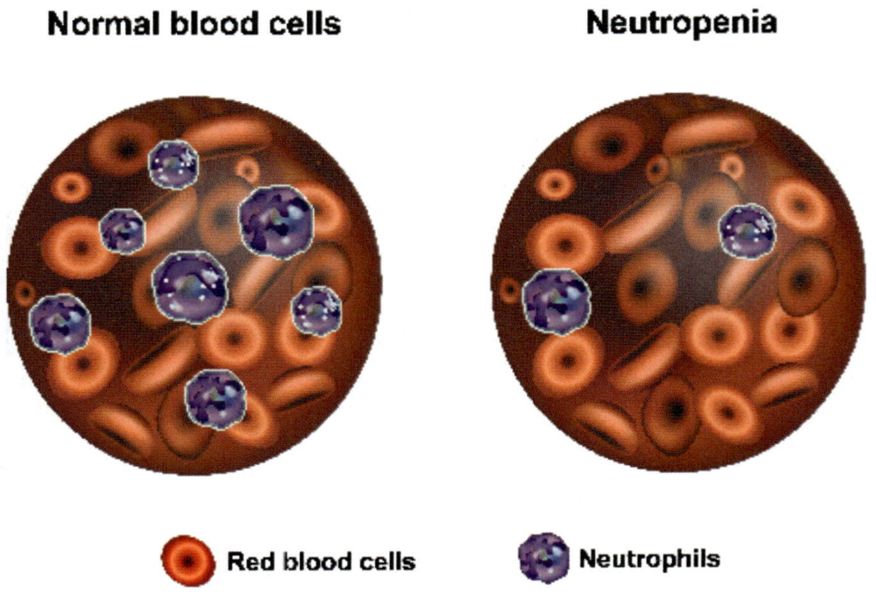

carefully watch for signs and symptoms of infection.

Signs and symptoms of infection may include:

- Fever (temperature of 100.4°F or 38°C and higher)
- Sore throat, sores in the mouth, or a toothache
- Abdominal pain
- Pain near the butt or when peeing
- Diarrhea
- Cough or shortness of breath
- Any redness, swelling, or pain around a cut, wound, or catheter

Bone pain

Bone pain is a common side effect of G-CSFs. It is not clear why. It may be due to the body's inflammatory response, which is how your immune system responds to infection.

Speak to your care team if you experience bone pain. They may be able to prescribe medication to relieve the pain.

What is febrile neutropenia?

When someone with neutropenia also develops a fever, it's called febrile neutropenia. With febrile neutropenia, your risk of infection may be higher than normal. This is because having fewer white blood cells leads to a reduced ability to fight infections, and your body is already compromised.

Preventive treatment

Before you receive chemotherapy or a bone marrow transplant, you may be given medicine to help prevent complications that may occur. This medicine is called a granulocyte colony-stimulating factor, or G-CSF.

G-CSFs boost the production of your white blood cells. Increasing your white blood cells supercharges your immune system to protect you from chemotherapy complications more effectively.

If your doctor thinks a G-CSF may be helpful, it will usually be given as an injection starting 1 to 3 days after chemotherapy.

G-CSFs include the following medicines:

- Filgrastim (Neupogen)
- Tbo-filgrastim (Granix)
- Pegfilgrastim (Neulasta)
- Efbemalenograstim alfa-vuxw (Ryzneuta)
- Eflapegrastim-xnst (Rolvedon)

In addition to being used for chemotherapy, G-CSFs are used to treat severe febrile neutropenia caused by radiation treatment.

Before chemotherapy starts

You'll be evaluated for risk of developing febrile neutropenia before your first chemotherapy treatment and throughout your chemotherapy treatments.

Cancer type

Your cancer type will be considered when discussing your risk for neutropenia. For example, neutropenia is a common side effect in people with leukemia but may not be as common in people with other cancers.

Dose and type of chemotherapy

Chemotherapy kills fast-growing cells throughout the body, including cancer cells and healthy cells. Your risk of febrile neutropenia may be increased based on the dose of chemotherapy or the chemotherapy regimen (combination of drugs) you receive.

Chemotherapy doses include:

- **High-dose chemotherapy** is an intense drug treatment. It can destroy bone marrow and cause severe side effects. Having a hematopoietic cell transplant is common after high-dose chemotherapy.
- **Dose-dense chemotherapy** is chemotherapy that's given more frequently than normally scheduled, with less time between doses. The purpose of the shortened time between doses is to kill as many of the cancer cells as possible.
- **Standard-dose chemotherapy** is given on a regular schedule, such as monthly. Certain combinations of chemotherapy drugs, even if they are not high dose or dose dense, can increase the risk of severe neutropenia.

Goal of treatment

Work with your care team to define your treatment goal. Your options will vary between cure or palliative care. Palliative care refers to relieving the side effects of chemotherapy, radiation treatment, or the symptoms of the disease. It's sometimes referred to as supportive care.

Patient risk factors

A risk factor is anything that increases your chances of disease. Your risk factors will be considered when deciding on your best course of treatment. Risk factors for neutropenia complications include age; other health concerns, such as lung or heart disease; and previous cancer treatments received.

Before starting chemotherapy, you'll be placed into a risk group based on your specific risk factors.

Your risk for developing febrile neutropenia will be based on:

- Your type of cancer or disease
- The type of chemotherapy planned
- If you have other serious health issues
- The goal of treatment (whether it is to cure the cancer or lessen symptoms)

After your risk is determined, you'll be placed into one of the following groups:

- Low risk
- Intermediate risk
- High risk

Low risk

If you are on a standard-dose chemotherapy regimen, don't have any symptoms, and have no other major health issues, then you are at low risk for febrile neutropenia. A low risk means you have less than a 1 in 10 chance of developing febrile neutropenia. Preventive treatment is not needed.

You'll be re-evaluated for febrile neutropenia after your first cycle of chemotherapy. If your risk does not change, you'll be tested for any changes to your risk score after each chemotherapy treatment.

Intermediate risk

If you are on a dose-dense chemotherapy regimen and have one or more of the risk factors listed in **Guide 2**, you are at intermediate risk. Intermediate risk means you have a 1 or 2 in 10 chance of developing febrile neutropenia.

You may receive G-CSFs if you're told you have intermediate risk.

High risk

If you are at high risk for febrile neutropenia, you have more than a 2 in 10 chance of developing it. This means you are on a high-dose chemotherapy regimen and have multiple risk factors listed in **Guide 2**, along with neutropenia.

High-risk febrile neutropenia will be treated with G-CSFs before your first chemotherapy cycle. You'll also be assessed after each chemotherapy cycle to determine if there are any changes and if further treatment for febrile neutropenia is necessary.

Guide 2
Intermediate febrile neutropenia risk

Risk factors	If...		Then...
• Prior chemotherapy or radiation therapy • Persistent neutropenia • Bone marrow involvement by tumor • Recent surgery and/or open wounds • Liver dysfunction • Renal dysfunction • 65 years of age or above and receiving full chemotherapy dose intensity	You have no risk factors	→	You will be observed
	You have one or more risk factors	→	You may receive G-CSFs

Febrile neutropenia during treatment

Sometimes people develop febrile neutropenia during chemotherapy. This might happen despite preventive treatment with G-CSFs.

If you're at risk for developing an infection-related complication, you may be treated with myeloid growth factors (MGFs).

MGFs are used to increase the number of blood cells and prevent infections. They're a larger category and can include G-CSFs or granulocyte-macrophage colony-stimulating factors (GM-CSFs).

Unlike G-CSFs, GM-CSFs stimulate the production of macrophages as well as granulocytes. These are both different kinds of white blood cells that can help fight infection in your body.

For more information on when MGFs and G-CSFs are used, see **Guide 3**.

If you received G-CSFs

Febrile neutropenia will be treated based on the drug received.

If you received filgrastim (Neupogen) or TBO-filgrastim (Granix), you'll continue this treatment.

If you were treated with pegfilgrastim (Neulasta), eflapegrastim-xnst (Rolvedon), or efbemalenograstim alfa-vuxw (Ryzneuta), no additional treatment with G-CSFs is recommended.

Guide 3
Therapeutic use of myeloid growth factors: Febrile neutropenia

	If...		Then...
Receiving or received preventive G-CSFs	You're receiving daily filgrastim or tbo-filgrastim	→	Continue G-CSFs
	You've received long-lasting pegfilgrastim	→	No additional G-CSFs
Did not receive preventive G-CSFs	You don't have risk factors for an infection-associated complication	→	No therapeutic MGFs
	You have risk factors present for an infection-associated complication	→	Therapeutic MGFs

Key points

- Neutropenia is a low white blood cell count. A low number of white blood cells reduces the body's ability to fight infections.
- Neutropenia is common after receiving chemotherapy. This is because chemotherapy kills cancer cells as well as healthy white blood cells.
- Most people who have neutropenia are not aware of it. People often find out when they have a blood test performed for other reasons.
- When someone with neutropenia also develops a fever, it is called febrile neutropenia. You may receive treatment to try to prevent febrile neutropenia.
- Febrile neutropenia is a serious condition. Any fever symptoms you experience should be reported to your care team as soon as possible.

We want your feedback!

Our goal is to provide helpful and easy-to-understand information on cancer. Take our survey to let us know what we got right and what we could do better.
NCCN.org/patients/feedback

Questions to ask

- Am I at risk for developing febrile neutropenia?
- Should I expect any side effects from treatment for neutropenia?
- What steps can I take to prevent infection while I have neutropenia?

5
Treating thrombocytopenia

Platelets are an important part of blood. They work with proteins called clotting factors to control bleeding inside our bodies and on our skin.

Platelets are made in your bone marrow along with white and red blood cells. They travel through your blood vessels and stick together (clot) to stop bleeding when needed.

What is thrombocytopenia?

Thrombocytopenia is when your blood has fewer platelets than normal. During thrombocytopenia, serious bleeding can occur inside your body or under your skin.

Thrombocytopenia can last for days to years depending on its cause. Many factors can cause thrombocytopenia, including:

- Bone marrow does not make enough platelets, like in leukemia, or other blood disorders, like hemophilia
- Infections, such as hepatitis C virus, HIV, or Epstein-Barr virus
- Certain drugs, such as warfarin (Coumadin), heparin, certain antibiotics, quinine, and chemotherapy drugs as well as drinking too much alcohol
- Platelets become trapped in the spleen (this happens in cirrhosis, myelofibrosis, and Gaucher disease)
- Red blood cell transfusions can thin platelet numbers in the blood
- The body may destroy or use up platelets made in the bone marrow. This occurs in many disorders, including immune thrombocytopenia, thrombotic thrombocytopenic purpura, and hemolytic-uremic syndrome

Let your care team know of any medicines you're currently taking that might make thrombocytopenia worse, like warfarin.

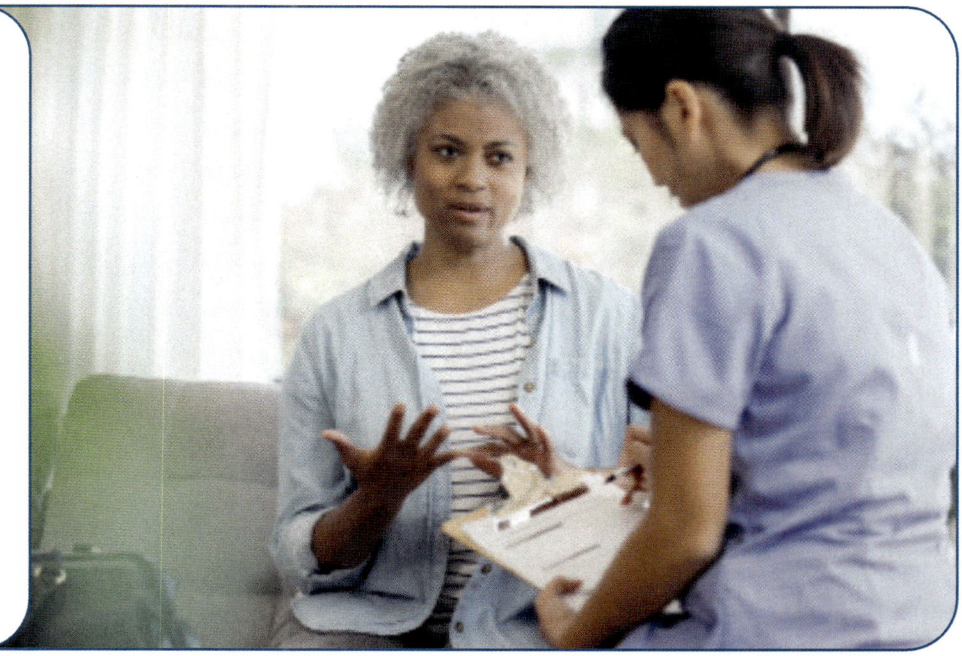

Treatment for thrombocytopenia

Treatment for thrombocytopenia depends on its cause. If you are found to have chemotherapy-induced thrombocytopenia, or CIT, you can expect to be treated with one or more of the following:

- Changing your chemotherapy dose or treatment
- Platelet transfusion
- Clinical trial of thrombopoietin receptor agonists (TPO-RAs)
- Romiplostim

Changing your chemotherapy

Chemotherapy destroys rapidly forming cells, such as blood or cancer cells. As a result, people treated with chemotherapy are more likely to have health problems related to low blood counts, like thrombocytopenia.

If your chemotherapy treatment is causing issues with low platelet count, your chemotherapy may be reduced or changed. Ask your care team to help you weigh the pros and cons of changing or delaying chemotherapy doses.

Platelet transfusion

You may receive a platelet transfusion if your platelet count is low. A platelet transfusion is used to stop or prevent bleeding in someone with thrombocytopenia.

During a transfusion, platelets are given through an intravenous (IV) drip with a needle placed into your arm. The platelets will be from 1 or more donors. The transfusion normally takes about 15 to 30 minutes to complete.

You can expect an immediate increase in the number of platelets in your blood after a transfusion.

For some, however, the effects may only be temporary (3–5 days), and more transfusions may be needed.

Thrombopoietin receptor agonists

The standard of care for thrombocytopenia is thrombopoietin receptor agonists, or TPO-RAs.

TPO-RAs raise platelet counts, decrease uncontrolled bleeding, and reduce the need for rescue treatments. Rescue treatments are given when standard therapy hasn't worked. An example of a TPO-RA is eltrombopag (Promacta).

Romiplostim

Romiplostim (Nplate) is a drug used to increase the number of platelets and decrease the risk of bleeding. It's a myeloid growth factor, or MGF, that's given as an injection. An MGF stimulates the bone marrow to make more stem cells.

After a stem cell transplant

You may develop thrombocytopenia after undergoing a hematopoietic cell transplant, or HCT. The goal of HCT is to cure cancer by replacing unhealthy cells with healthy ones.

Also called a stem cell transplant or a bone marrow transplant, an HCT destroys cancer cells in the bone marrow and replaces them with new, healthy blood cells from a donor.

These healthy, blood-forming stem cells are infused through a needle. These new cells travel to the bone marrow, where they'll grow and make new healthy blood cells. They may also recognize and attack any remaining cancer cells.

Testing

If you develop thrombocytopenia after an HCT, you'll be tested for:

- Nutritional deficiencies
- Medications and supplements that reduce platelet production
- Infection
- Immune thrombocytopenia
- HCT failure (the transplant didn't work)
- Transplanted cells attacking the body's immune cells
- Cancer recurrence (comes back)

Treatment

If you have thrombocytopenia after an HCT, your doctor will try to determine the cause.

If there is no clear cause, the following thrombocytopenia treatments are options:

- Platelet transfusion
- Clinical trial of TPO-RAs
- Eltrombopag

Key points

- Platelets are an important part of blood. They control bleeding inside our bodies and on our skin.
- Thrombocytopenia occurs when your immune system attacks the platelets in your blood.
- During thrombocytopenia, serious bleeding can occur inside your body or under your skin.
- If you have chemotherapy-induced thrombocytopenia, treatment options include platelet transfusion, reduction in chemotherapy, romiplostim, or a clinical trial.
- A hematopoietic cell transplant (HCT) destroys cells in the bone marrow and replaces them with new, healthy, blood-forming cells from another person.

Questions to ask

- Are there any restrictions to my day-to-day life while I have thrombocytopenia?
- What's the risk of my bone marrow transplant causing thrombocytopenia?
- Can I do anything to reduce my risk of thrombocytopenia bleeding events?

6

ICAHT and supportive care

ICAHT, or immune effector cell-associated hematologic toxicity, is a life-threatening side effect of some cancer treatments. This complication causes neutropenia, anemia, and thrombocytopenia all at once.

Immune effector cell-associated hematologic toxicity, or ICAHT, may seem like a lot to read. Put simply, it's a side effect of some cancer treatments where the body develops all 3 types of low blood cell counts at once. This can be life-threatening, but NCCN experts have devised guidelines to help prevent ICAHT where possible, described in this chapter.

Guide 4
Risk factors for ICAHT

You have cancer in your bone marrow
You have many cancerous tumors
You have anemia, thrombocytopenia, or neutropenia
You're already inflamed
You have an active infection
You have had a bone marrow transplant
You have had bridging therapy (anticoagulant medications like warfarin [Coumadin])
Your CAR-HEMATOTOX score is 2 or higher

Evaluating ICAHT risk

Before you begin treatment with an immune effector cell therapy, such as chimeric antigen receptor (CAR) T-cell therapy, your care team will evaluate your risk for ICAHT. These risk factors are listed in **Guide 4**.

A CAR-HEMATOTOX score determines your level of risk of neutropenia based on the chemicals that exist in your blood, such as ferritin.

Treating ICAHT

Treatment of ICAHT is determined based on how many of the risk factors in the previous section you have. If you have none of the risk factors discussed in the "Evaluating ICAHT risk" section, you might receive granulocyte-colony stimulating factors (G-CSFs) to prevent febrile neutropenia.

See *Chapter 4: Neutropenia* for more information on G-CSFs and febrile neutropenia.

If you have any risk factors discussed in the previous section, then you will receive G-CSFs 2 days or later than the initial treatment of CAR T-cell therapy. If there's no response within a week or so, you might receive stem cells or thrombopoietin receptor agonists (TPO-RAs). See *Chapter 5: Thrombocytopenia* for more information about TPO-RAs.

The low blood cell counts (neutropenia, anemia, and thrombocytopenia) caused by ICAHT are each treated as previously described in other chapters.

Supportive care for low blood cell counts

Supportive care is an important part of cancer care. The goal is to improve your quality of life during and after cancer treatment, including treatment for low blood cell counts. Supportive care is for everyone with cancer and their families, not just for those at the end of life. It's also known as palliative care.

Supportive care includes a wide range of services. Supportive care prevents or manages the symptoms of cancer and the side effects of cancer treatment, like pain and cancer-related fatigue. It also addresses the mental, social, emotional, and spiritual concerns faced by people with cancer.

Supportive care provides help with additional needs, such as:

- Making treatment decisions
- Coordinating your care
- Paying for care
- Planning for advance care and end of life

Read more about the types of support you may receive in *NCCN Guidelines for Patients: Palliative Care*, available at NCCN.org/patientguidelines and on the NCCN Patient Guides for Cancer app.

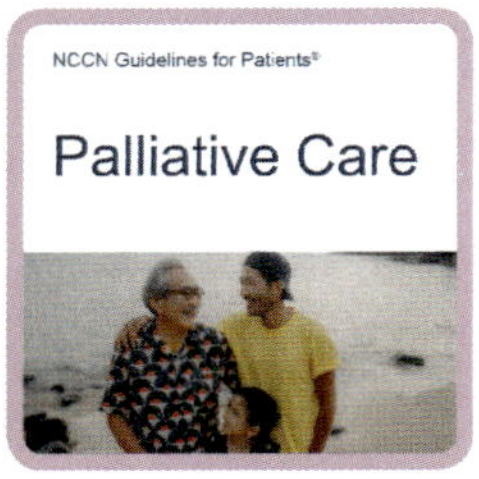

"People will ask how they can help. Be specific. You can cook for me. Please pack meals in 4-ounce containers because that is all I can handle at any one time."

Key points

- ICAHT, or immune effector cell-associated hematologic toxicity, is a life-threatening complication of some cancer treatments.
- Your risk level determines what sort of treatment you require. If you have more than 1 risk factor, you will receive G-CSF treatment.
- Low blood cell counts caused by ICAHT are treated as needed using the treatments listed in previous chapters.
- Supportive care is always available if you need it. It's not just for end-of-life care.

Questions to ask

- If I'm receiving a CAR T-cell therapy, what is my risk for ICAHT?
- What can I do to help make sure that my blood cell counts stay at the correct level?
- Can I receive supportive care to help ease my pain?
- Can I receive financial assistance or psychosocial support at this time?

What's next?

The best defense against low blood counts is to be an active participant in your care. Talk to your care team and let them know how you're feeling during all stages of your cancer treatment journey. No question is too simple, no comment is a complaint.

You are your best ally in this journey.

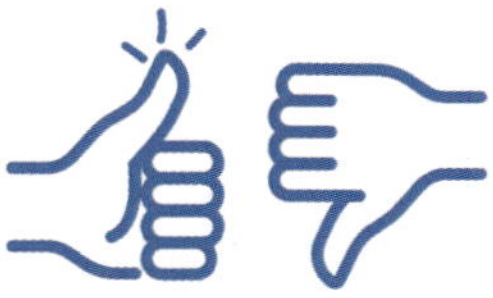

Let us know what you think!

Please take a moment to complete an online survey about the NCCN Guidelines for Patients.
NCCN.org/patients/response

7 Other resources

Want to learn more? Here's how you can get additional help.

What else to know

This guide helps you know your options so you can make informed decisions and improve your cancer care. But it's not the only resource that you have.

Ask for as much information and help as you need. Many people are interested in learning more about:

- The details of cytopenias and their symptoms
- Being part of a care team
- Getting financial help
- Finding a cancer care professional who's an expert in their field
- Coping with other health problems

What else to do

Your health care center can help you with next steps. It often has on-site resources to help meet your needs and find answers to your questions. Health care centers can also inform you of resources in your community.

In addition to help from your providers, the resources listed in the next section provide support for many people like yourself.

Where to get help

Look through the list below and visit the provided websites to learn more about these organizations.

Blood Cancer United
Bloodcancerunited.org

Cancer*Care*
cancercare.org

Imerman Angels
Imermanangels.org

Leukemia Research Foundation
Leukemiarf.org

NMDP
Nmdp.org

Triage Cancer
triagecancer.org

Questions to ask

- What will happen if I do nothing?
- How do my age, health, and other factors affect my options?
- Am I a candidate for a blood stem cell transplant?
- Am I a candidate for a clinical trial?
- Which option is proven to work best for my type, age, and other risk factors?

Words to know

anemia
A condition in which the number of red blood cells is low.

blood smear
A test in which a drop of blood is placed on a slide and viewed with a microscope to assess the size, shape, type, and maturity of the blood cells.

blood stem cell
An immature blood-forming cell from which all other types of blood cells are made. Also called hematopoietic stem cell.

bone marrow
The soft, sponge-like tissue in the center of most bones where blood cells are made.

chemotherapy
Treatment with drugs that kill abnormal cells or stop new ones from being made.

complete blood count (CBC)
A test of the number of blood cells in a sample.

donor
A person who gives their organs, tissues, or cells to another person.

erythropoiesis-stimulating agent (ESA)
A drug that tells (stimulates) the bone marrow to make more red blood cells.

erythropoietin
A substance that is made naturally in the body and that tells (stimulates) the bone marrow to make more red blood cells.

fatigue
Severe tiredness despite getting enough sleep, which limits the ability to function.

febrile neutropenia
Fever during a period of having a significantly low white blood cell count.

granulocyte colony-stimulating factor (G-CSF)
A substance that helps (stimulates) the bone marrow to make more white blood cells called neutrophils. It is made naturally in the body but can also be made in a lab.

hematopoiesis
The production of blood cells and platelets that occurs in the bone marrow.

hematopoietic stem cell or hematopoietic cell
An immature blood-forming cell from which all other types of blood cells are made. Also called blood stem cell.

hemoglobin
A protein in red blood cells that carries oxygen.

hormone
A chemical in the body that activates cells or organs.

immune system
The body's natural defense against infection and disease.

iron
A mineral found in red blood cells that the body needs to make new red blood cells.

mean corpuscular volume
The average size of your red blood cells.

myeloid growth factors (MGFs)
Molecules that play important roles in the growth, survival, and differentiation of blood progenitor cells, as well as in the functional activation of mature cells.

neutropenia
A condition in which the number of white blood cells, called neutrophils, is low.

neutrophil
A type of white blood cell that helps fight infections and has small particles (granules).

platelet
A type of blood cell that helps control bleeding.

red blood cell
A type of blood cell that carries oxygen from the lungs to the rest of the body.

red blood cell transfusion
Slow injection of red blood cells into a vein.

regimen
A treatment plan that specifies the dose, schedule, and duration of treatment.

reticulocyte
Younger (precursor) cells that become mature red blood cells.

transfusion
Slow injection of whole blood (red blood cells, white blood cells, and platelets) or parts of blood into a vein.

white blood cell
A type of blood cell that helps fight infections in the body.

share with us.

Take our survey and help make the NCCN Guidelines for Patients better for everyone!

NCCN.org/patients/comments

NCCN Contributors

This patient guide is based on the NCCN Clinical Practice Guidelines in Oncology (NCCN Guidelines®) for Hematopoietic Growth Factors, Version 3.2026. It was adapted, reviewed, and published with help from the following people:

Dorothy A. Shead, MS
Senior Director
Patient Information Operations

Tim Rinehart, MS
Medical Writer

Lisa Diehl
Production Layout Artist

The NCCN Clinical Practice Guidelines in Oncology (NCCN Guidelines®) for Hematopoietic Growth Factors, Version 3.2026 were developed by the following NCCN Panel Members:

*Elizabeth A. Griffiths, MD/Chair
Roswell Park Comprehensive Cancer Center

Mark Geyer, MD/Vice-Chair
Memorial Sloan Kettering Cancer Center

Iman Ahmed, PharmD
University of Michigan Rogel Cancer Center

Samia Asif, MBBS
Fred & Pamela Buffett Cancer Center

Kimo Bachiashvili, MD
O'Neal Comprehensive Cancer Center at UAB

*John Baird, MD
City of Hope National Medical Center

Shivani Bakhshi, DO
Abramson Cancer Center at the University of Pennsylvania

Emily Chheng, PharmD, BCOP
Case Comprehensive Cancer Center/ University Hospitals Seidman Cancer Center and Cleveland Clinic Taussig Cancer Institute

Rita Cool, PharmD, BCOP
The University of Texas MD Anderson Cancer Center

Tyler Dickerson, PharmD, BCOP
The Ohio State University Comprehensive Cancer Center - James Cancer Hospital and Solove Research Institute

Shira Dinner, MD
Robert H. Lurie Comprehensive Cancer Center of Northwestern University

Michael Fallon, PharmD
University of Wisconsin Carbone Cancer Center

John Glaspy, MD, MPH
UCLA Jonsson Comprehensive Cancer Center

Ivana Gojo, MD
Johns Hopkins Kimmel Cancer Center

*Khushali Jhaveri, MD
Indiana University Melvin and Bren Simon Comprehensive Cancer Center

Wajih Zaheer Kidwai, MD
Yale Cancer Center/ Smilow Cancer Hospital

Yuchen Liu, MD
Robert H. Lurie Comprehensive Cancer Center of Northwestern University

Gary H. Lyman, MD, MPH
Fred Hutchinson Cancer Center

Anjlee Mahajan, MD
UC Davis Comprehensive Cancer Center

*Ginny Mason, BSN, RN
Inflammatory Breast Cancer Research Foundation

Victoria Nachar, PharmD, BCOP
University of Michigan Rogel Cancer Center

Anthony Nguyen, MD
UC San Diego Moores Cancer Center

Thomas Odeny, MD, PhD, MPH
Siteman Cancer Center at Barnes-Jewish Hospital and Washington University School of Medicine

Sukhmani Padda, MD
Fox Chase Cancer Center

Hetalkumari Patel, PharmD, BCOP
UT Southwestern Simmons Comprehensive Cancer Center

Shiven Patel, MD, MBA
Huntsman Cancer Institute at the University of Utah

Lia E. Perez, MD
Moffitt Cancer Center

Fauzia Riaz, MD
Stanford Cancer Institute

Kelley Rone, DNP, APRN
Mayo Clinic Comprehensive Cancer Center

Rachel Rosovsky, MD, MPH
Mass General Cancer Center

Martha Wadleigh, MD
Dana-Farber/Brigham and Women's Cancer Center

*Kelly Westbrook, MD
Duke Cancer Institute

Bradley Yelvington, PharmD, BCOP
Vanderbilt-Ingram Cancer Center

Benjamin Yoder, PharmD, BCOP
University of Colorado Cancer Center

NCCN

Frankie Jones
Guidelines Coordinator

Swathi Ramakrishnan, PhD
Oncology Scientist/Medical Writer

* Reviewed this patient guide. For disclosures, visit NCCN.org/disclosures.

NCCN Cancer Centers

For contact information visit NCCN.org/cancercenters.

Abramson Cancer Center
at the University of Pennsylvania
Philadelphia, Pennsylvania

Case Comprehensive Cancer Center/
University Hospitals Seidman Cancer Center and
Cleveland Clinic Taussig Cancer Institute
Cleveland, Ohio

City of Hope National Medical Center
Duarte, California

Dana-Farber/Brigham and Women's Cancer Center |
Mass General Cancer Center
Boston, Massachusetts

Duke Cancer Institute
Durham, North Carolina

Fox Chase Cancer Center
Philadelphia, Pennsylvania

Fred & Pamela Buffett Cancer Center
Omaha, Nebraska

Fred Hutchinson Cancer Center
Seattle, Washington

Huntsman Cancer Institute at the University of Utah
Salt Lake City, Utah

Indiana University Melvin and Bren Simon
Comprehensive Cancer Center
Indianapolis, Indiana

Johns Hopkins Kimmel Cancer Center
Baltimore, Maryland

Mayo Clinic Comprehensive Cancer Center
Phoenix/Scottsdale, Arizona
Jacksonville, Florida
Rochester, Minnesota

Memorial Sloan Kettering Cancer Center
New York, New York

Moffitt Cancer Center
Tampa, Florida

O'Neal Comprehensive Cancer Center at UAB
Birmingham, Alabama

Robert H. Lurie Comprehensive Cancer Center
of Northwestern University
Chicago, Illinois

Roswell Park Comprehensive Cancer Center
Buffalo, New York

Siteman Cancer Center at Barnes-Jewish Hospital
and Washington University School of Medicine
St. Louis, Missouri

St. Jude Children's Research Hospital/
The University of Tennessee Health Science Center
Memphis, Tennessee

Stanford Cancer Institute
Stanford, California

The Ohio State University Comprehensive Cancer Center -
James Cancer Hospital and Solove Research Institute
Columbus, Ohio

The UChicago Medicine Comprehensive Cancer Center
Chicago, Illinois

The University of Texas MD Anderson Cancer Center
Houston, Texas

UC Davis Comprehensive Cancer Center
Sacramento, California

UC San Diego Moores Cancer Center
La Jolla, California

UCLA Jonsson Comprehensive Cancer Center
Los Angeles, California

UCSF Helen Diller Family Comprehensive Cancer Center
San Francisco, California

University of Colorado Cancer Center
Aurora, Colorado

University of Michigan Rogel Cancer Center
Ann Arbor, Michigan

University of Wisconsin Carbone Cancer Center
Madison, Wisconsin

UT Southwestern Simmons
Comprehensive Cancer Center
Dallas, Texas

Vanderbilt-Ingram Cancer Center
Nashville, Tennessee

Yale Cancer Center/Smilow Cancer Hospital
New Haven, Connecticut

Notes

Index

Made in the USA
Coppell, TX
22 August 2026

87830620R00029